Pregnancy:

Childbirth, Motherhood and Nutrition – Everything You NEED to Know When Having a Baby

I0468073

Table of Contents

-

Free Bonus!!!

We would like to offer you our FREE Guide to jump start you on a path to improve your life & Exclusive access to our Breakthrough Book Club!!! It's a place where we offer a NEW FREE E-book every week! Also our members are actively discussing, reviewing, and sharing their thoughts on the Book of The Week and on topics to help each other Breakthrough Life's Obstacles! With a Chance to win a $25 Gift Card EVERY Month! Please Enjoy Your FREE Guide & Access to the **Breakthrough Book Club**

https://publishfs.leadpages.co/the-breakthrough-book-club-d/

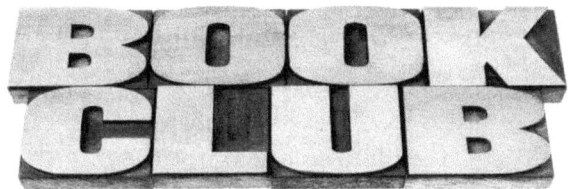

Introduction

In the fast-paced, high-powered world of today, thinking about starting a family is no easy thing. Both partners must sit and have open discussions about whether they want to have children, how many kids they would like to have and then go about planning accordingly.

For women in particular, the decision is a lot more multifaceted than simply deciding to have a child and then fixing up financials and the like for it. Given that you will be carrying a child within you for close to ten full months, your body will undergo drastic changes that will affect you even after you bring your baby into this world. As such, it is not a decision to be made lightly; having open and honest discussions with your partner goes a long way in helping you make up your mind.

But once you *have* made that choice – or you're very seriously considering taking the plunge into motherhood – what you need the most is advice! From pregnancy to childbirth oto post-natal care for both yourself and your baby, preparing to bring your own bundle of joy home is a journey filled with ups and downs and more hiccups that we can count with our hands! It can be a very frightening thing, especially for first-timers, and every little piece of information you can get your hands on will make you sleep that much better at night!

If you are an expecting mother, or you want to know mother about pregnancy and childbirth before you conceive a baby – you have come to the right place! In this book, I will help you explore the intricacies of being pregnant and looking after yourself and your child before, during and after your pregnancy! The world of child rearing and caring is vast and massive; this book will get you started with the basics of what you need to know!

Thank you for choosing this book and I hope you find it informative!

Chapter 1: Talking to Your Partner About Having a Baby

So you think you want to bring a baby into the world... or pregnancy has made the choice for you. Now you need to take time to think about what all you need to talk about. There are things you might not have ever thought about talking about. You shouldn't wait to bring things up because if it was not planned the longer you wait to tell your partner you could start an argument. If you end up fighting because of it and realize that you are not what you thought you were together it could leave you taking care of both sides of the responsibility.

This could have been a little drastic, but there are things that need to be agreed on before pregnancy. If it happens before you get to talk about this you really need to talk about what is going to happen and it should happen early on in case things go bad. Here is a list of 15 things that need to be agreed on by you and your partner when thinking about having a baby.

15 Things You Should Consider Before Becoming Pregnant

How you want to birth

If you want to have a home birth and this is a problem for your partner because he doesn't want his gaming couch to get stuff on it, your partner and you need to talk. Your partner should be okay with the way you want to birth and the methods. It may help to practice for giving labor. Your partner should be your number one supporter and if he needs to there are parental classes he can take. You don't want to get to the final stretch and your partner not want to go along with the plan.

Potential complications

The what ifs are something that you should always discuss even if no one wants to, but try not to go overboard. What if your child is special needs? How would you take care of the child together? What if you have a complicated pregnancy? It is important to go over these topics but you should only go over them in more detail if you know that you will experience it beforehand.

Circumcision

You or you and your partner need to decide if your male child should be circumcised or not.

Name choice

You may want a name that is more unique and your partner may want something that is popular. This can be a very difficult decision, but you have 9 months to come up with one. There are ways that you can narrow these down and get a little of what you want and a little of what he wants so that both of you are satisfied.

Vaccinations

Both you and your partner need to read about vaccinations and discuss your thoughts on these.

Conquering bad habits

Smoking is a bad habit but maybe your partner doesn't want to quit. This is something else that you should discuss together.

Money

Money is an important thing to talk about and if this does not cause a fight with your partner than that is great. Children take a lot of money to care for and it is good to put money to the side.

Breastfeeding

Your partner needs to support you by keeping you hydrated while   breastfeeding.

Religion

You and your partner may have 2 different faiths. You should discuss what religion you will want your child to incorporate into their life. There are many ways that couples could want things to go for this so make sure to talk about it now.

Discipline

Just like any mother, you do not want your toddler having a tantrum that you are not able to discipline without facing disapproval from your partner. Before your baby enters this world, you should ensure that you and your partner are on the same wavelength when it comes to discipline in common situations.

Food

As your baby gets older and heads off to grandmas for visits, chances are that grandma will fill her full of cookies at lunch time and tons of sugary drinks, including soda. If this is something that you do not want, but your partner doesn't mind, this can become a problem. It is even worse when your partner behaves like grandma and does the same exact thing.

Breakdown of Responsibilities

Will dad work and mom stay home, or will it be the other way around? If both of you plan to work, what will you do about child care?

To Cut or Not to Cut: Cutting Your child's hair (boy or girl) – Whether it seems like a big deal now, cutting of hair is a major battle point in any household with children. Should their hair be long, sort? – doesn't sound like a complicated dilemma, but in many houses, it can become a highly contested battlefield.

Co Sleeping

Co sleeping as a newborn may be a given. However, some mothers tend to extend co sleeping into childhood. While co sleeping into childhood is inconvenient, it does not mean that you will never have sex again, it just means that there will be a third person snuggling afterward.

Taking a Break from Sex, Can your Partner Handle it?

After having a baby, enjoying the sheer and utter exhaustion through the first six to eight weeks, and checking on your baby every 20 minutes after they move to the nursery, some parents lose their sex drive. Many people think that it is just women who suffer from this. The truth is that men suffer from loss of sex drive as well. Because of this, there must be a lot of patience on the part of both parents. Even if there is a lull in your sex life, things will turn around soon. Who knows, your sex life could turn out better than ever.

Are Both Partners Ready?

Maybe you and your partner have never discussed having a baby, your you said you wanted kids at some point or another. Maybe you and your partner agreed that you should have your first child when you turn 25. Now that the time has come, one of you are ready to start creating a family – and the other partner is having serious reservations.

Hesitation about leaping into parenthood is more common than you may think, according to. Many psychoanalysts, sees many couples in his practice that are on the brink of having a child, but one person in the relationship has serious reservations. They are worried, or wonder what the hurry is.

Many psychoanalysts have noted several times that when one person is suddenly desperate to have a baby, the urge may have more to do with an unstable marriage than actually wanting to become a parent. In these cases, the partner who has become desperate is making an attempt to solidify a relationship that has stumbled onto shaky ground. They feel that having a baby will bring their spouse closer and build a deeper relationship.

Many believe that having a baby will help restore the strong trust and intimacy that the relationship is now lacking.

If the baby was previously planned and one of the relationship partners begins blocking the thought, there could be more at stake than just having a baby. Many times, this hesitation revolves around child hood issues. This means that the hesitant partner might need to deal with other issues they faced in childhood that were unresolved. These could be unresolved issues surrounding their childhood, issues about his or her own parents, or trauma they suffered as a child.

How do you figure out what is going on, and determine the next step?

The True Problem – Getting to the Root

Some concerns, like the size of your house and financial issues are not the main reasons your partner is behaving this way. Lack of time, not enough money, not enough space ... these are all fabricated concepts that people use to draw attention from the true reasons they are not ready for a baby.

The partner who has the concerns must break through the excuses to locate the real reasons they are not ready for a child and come to an understanding of the true reason they are resisting a baby at this time. This may, or may not, be an issue that the couple needs to approach together. Typically, the partner who is resistant needs a neutral, safe person to talk to about their feelings, and someone who will not judge them based on their past.

Chapter 2: Prenatal Care

The term prenatal care is a very broad expression that covers the entire gamut of your pregnancy care, right up until when your child is born. Ideally, prenatal care begins even *before* you become pregnant – you should begin taking special care of yourself and your body three months before you start trying to conceive.

Once you have made the decision that you want to enter into motherhood, there a few things you must practice regularly –

- Stop smoking; reduce your alcohol intake

- Start taking folic acid supplements

- Avoid getting into touch with any toxic chemicals or materials

- Pay regular visits to your doctor to make sure you are healthy and safe

For those women who have difficulty getting pregnant, regular visits to your doctor are a must. The cases of women with polycystic ovaries and the like are increasing regularly; for such women, getting pregnant can be a challenge, though it is certainly not impossible. Listen to what your doctor tells you and follow all rules to the letter – soon, you will find yourself glowing and happy with child!

Once you have confirmed that you *are*, indeed, pregnant, you need to get into the groove of things! The first thing to do, of course, is consulting your OB-GYN and schedule your regular appointments, from ultrasounds to blood screenings. Print out this list and hang it up on your refrigerator or white board where you will get to see it every day – that way, you will never miss an appointment and end up neglecting care for your baby!

In case you haven't found yourself a good caregiver yet, start looking straight away! Finding the perfect midwife or obstetrician to suit you and your needs can take time – don't postpone it. Consult close friends who have been through the process before and make a list of prospective doctors before you visit them one by one and then make your choice.

Now you need to slowly start making changes to your lifestyle so that you are well adjusted by the time baby makes its way into the world. The practical side of things begins with planning your financials and scheduling your maternity leave; for yourself, you will need to start by eating healthier and taking good care of yourself! Understand the changes your body will be experiencing in the next couple of months so that you are not frightened and can take care of yourself better.

Here are some quick things to add to your diet to get all these nutrients naturally.

- **For Folic Acid Requirements** – As I already mentioned, this an essential nutrient before conception and through the course of your pregnancy. Add it to your diet in the form of ½ cup of boiled spinach, ½ cup of boiled Great Northern Beans, 4 boiled Asparagus pieces, 1 orange, 1 ounce of dry, roasted peanuts, etc. Remember, you don't have to take *all* of these everyday; spread it over the week and make your diet healthy!

- **Iron Requirements** – This is possibly the most problematic nutrient in your body during pregnancy; your body expands the volume of blood it produces in order to help your baby make his/her entire blood supply as well. This means that you need iron for both you and the baby – too many pregnant women fall victim to anemia, thereby becoming fatigued too easily.

Eating lean red meat, poultry, fish, beans and other vegetables will greatly reduce your risk of anemia. Add ½ cup of boiled kidney beans, ½ cup of boiled spinach, 85g of roasted lean beef tenderloin, etc, to your daily diet so that you get adequate iron supplements. Remember – iron from animal products is most easily absorbed. To enhance absorption from plant sources, pair them up with a drink that is high in vitamin C, like orange juice or tomato juice. Keep in mind though, that calcium can decrease iron absorption, so drink juices that are not calcium-fortified.

- **For Calcium Requirements** – Needless to say, dairy products are your best source of calcium; other than dairy products, broccoli and kale are excellent calcium providers. Add 1-cup milk, 170g of low-fat fruit yogurt, 28g of mozzarella cheese, ½ cup of boiled spinach, etc, to your regular diet to get the supplements you need!

- **Vitamin D Requirements** – Vitamin D helps build your baby's bones and teeth; you're going to need to add fish to your diet, along with 1 cup of milk and 1 large, hard-boiled egg to your daily diet.

- **Protein Requirements** – Protein is crucial for

your baby's development, so include it in your daily diet in the form of lean meat, poultry, fish, dairy products, beans and peas. Take 1 cup of low-fat 1% milk cottage cheese, fish, ½ cup boiled lentils, 1 cup milk, 1 large, hard-boiled egg, etc, to ensure you get your daily protein quotient.

These are the most important nutrients you will need to add to your diet. Don't worry about having a perfect pregnancy diet – there is no such thing! There exists no magic formula; just make sure you're eating healthy, with a balance of all required nutrients, particularly the ones mentioned above. Consult your doctor before you take any extra supplements and keep them informed about your daily food intake as well!

Avoid alcohol when you're carrying a baby. It reaches your child through your bloodstream very quickly, so much so that your baby can end up with higher blood alcohol levels than you. Even if you take only one drink a day, you end up increasing your odd having a low birth weight baby and your child developing problems in speaking, learning, language, etc. Take more than one drink, and you risk your child developing fetal alcohol syndrome (FAS), which can lead to mental and growth retardation, heart defects and the like. Drinking also increases odds of stillbirth and miscarriage – so for the sake of a healthy, happy child, don't drink when pregnant!

It goes without saying that you also need to swear off any drug habit you may have. Cocaine restricts the blood flow to the uterus, leading to problems like miscarriage, placental abruption, premature delivery, stillbirth, etc. And if drugs are bad, smoking is equally horrible, leading to similar problems of miscarriage, placental abruption and the like. Stay away from drugs, alcohol and pot if you want to deliver a happy baby.

Another important thing to cut back on is caffeine. Avid coffee-drinkers, step away from that enticing morning coffee fix – it's been proven to increase your risk of miscarriage. It has no nutritive value as such and in fact, acts as a deterrent, making it harder for your body to absorb iron, which – as we already discussed – is essential for your baby's development.

Added to that is the fact that caffeine is a brilliant stimulant, which in this case, works against you – you may find it hard to get a good night's rest, which is essential for a good and happy pregnancy.

Switch to decaf if you can't swear off coffee completely; constantly check the caffeine content of any other products you consume, like tea or chocolate.

Also remember to drink *plenty* of water. Water is how the nutrients are carried to your baby; it prevents problems like constipation, hemorrhoids, too much swelling, urinary tract infections, etc. Drink too little water and you run the risk of premature labor. You need to drink a minimum of 10 cups of water in a day; add other fluids like juices and herbal (ginger or peppermint) tea.

Chapter 3: What to Eat

A well-balanced meal consists of quite a few elements. Your meal should consist of several elements in small amounts. This list will help you to create a balanced meal, every time.

Experts on pregnancy nutrition have spent years of study in order determine the right nutrition during this special time of a woman's life. A well-balanced diet that supports both the needs of the mother-to-be and the baby should basically include around 80-100 g of protein, water and salt, as well as enough calories from various food groups.

- 2 to 3 servings fish, meat, legumes or nuts, and tofu
- 1 serving of yellow vegetables
- 2 servings of green vegetables
- 2 to 3 servings of dairy such as milk, cheese, yogurt, eggs
- 3 servings of whole grain cereals, whole grain breads or other foods containing high-complex carbohydrates
- 3 servings of fruits
- 6 to 8 glasses of water clean, filtered
- Salt to taste

This list may seem like a lot but is actually just enough to supply the needed nutrients for both you and your baby.

Choosing Meats and Proteins While Pregnant

According to the WHO (World Health Organization), pregnant women should eat at least 75 grams of proteins per day. Studies have shown that at this minimum amount, a pregnant woman can already decrease the risk for diseases of pregnancy like pre-eclampsia or metabolic toxemia that develops during late pregnancy (in susceptible people).

Proteins have numerous functions in the body. However, getting the right amount every day is not the sole marker for a nutritious and well-balanced diet. It has to come from healthy sources. Choose lean meats from organically raised animals, such as free-range chicken and cattle. Remember, anything in the food you eat can affect your baby. Stay away from meats that come from animals that have been treated with loads of antibiotics. The antibiotics leave residue on the meats and will stay there until you eat them. These residues will cause problems in your body and may affect the baby as well. Also, animals that have not been raised organically may also have been treated with artificial hormones. This is a practice among some livestock growers to improve the yield of each meat producer. But these artificial hormones prove to be unhealthy for humans, most especially to pregnant women and their babies. These can seriously interfere with the baby's growth and development.

Best Sources of Protein

- Beef
- Poultry
- Turkey
- Fish
- Nuts
- Tofu
- Legumes

- Eggs
- Milk
- Soy cheese
- Cottage cheese
- Whole grain

Other Inexpensive Sources of Protein

- Eggs
- Milk
- Dairy products like cheese
- Beans
- Soy beans
- Soy products
- Nuts
- Yogurt
- Cheddar cheese
- Dark green leafy vegetables
- Canned fish (with the fish bones still intact)
- Almonds
- Sesame seeds
- Fish
- Fortified cereals and breads
- Fortified soy milk
- Fortified juices

Choosing Vegetables While Pregnant

Vegetables are powerhouses of nutrients, especially with

minerals and vitamins. Each vegetable contains not only 1 kind of nutrient but also a handful. The amounts vary but every vegetable contains most of the minerals and vitamins that you need.

Dark green vegetables are rich in carbohydrates, bulk fiber and water. They also contain heaps of minerals and vitamins like magnesium, vitamin C, iron, vitamin B, calcium and vitamin A. Darker-colored vegetables tend to have higher amounts of the nutrients you need on a daily basis.

The best way to get all the natural goodness of vegetables is to eat them raw. Heating can destroy the delicate minerals and vitamins. Steaming and baking are also good because these cooking methods do not alter these nutrients much.

Microwaving vegetables is one of the worst things you can do. Just a few short minutes in the microwave can deplete the minerals and vitamins in a vegetable to almost nothing. Other cooking methods tend to breakdown the nutrients so much that very little remains intact for the body to use.

Great Sources for Whole Grains

- Buckwheat groats (kasha)
- Quinoa
- Wild rice
- Brown rice
- Wheat germ
- Wheat gluten
- Whole wheat pasta

- Whole grain cereals
- Whole oats

Great Sources for Fruits

- Kiwi fruit
- Bananas
- Oranges
- Apples
- Pears
- Nectarines
- Plums
- Pears
- Cantaloupe
- Grapefruits
- Mango
- Peaches

Great Sources for Green vegetables

- Broccoli
- Dark green lettuce
- Lambs lettuce
- Asparagus
- Spinach
- Green beans
- Arugula
- Swiss chard
- Zucchini
- Kale

- Dairy
- Cottage cheese
- Hard cheese
- Yogurt
- Milk
- Eggs

Natural Sources of Folic acid

- Lentils
- Peas
- Dried beans
- Kidney beans
- Lima beans
- White beans
- Soybeans
- Dark green leafy vegetables such as asparagus, okra, collard greens, and broccoli
- Spinach
- Turnip greens
- Brussels sprouts
- Root vegetables
- Brewer's yeast
- Whole grains
- Bulgur wheat
- Wheat germ
- Salmon
- Organ meats
- Avocado
- Orange juice
- Milk

Natural Sources of Iron

- Stomach upset
- Constipation
- Abdominal discomfort
- Vomiting
- Nausea
- Heartburn
- Diarrhea (less common)

The recommended daily intake of iron is 27 mg. Foods rich in iron include:

- Pork
- Beef
- Organ meats
- Red meats
- Poultry
- Fish
- Blackstrap molasses
- Cherry juice
- Dried beans
- Dried fruits
- Spinach
- Oatmeal
- Wheat germ
- Grains fortified with iron

Other Important Vitamins for

Pregnancy

Important Vitamins for Pregnancy

Zinc

This is a very important mineral that you have to make sure you get in the right amounts throughout your pregnancy. Zinc supports normal fetal development, such as the formation of the immune system and the components of the blood. Zinc improves birth weight, which is an important indicator of newborn health.

The recommended daily intake of zinc is 11 to 12 mg. it helps in the production of enzymes and insulin. Great natural sources include:

- Dairy products
- Red meats
- Whole grains
- Nuts
- Squash seeds
- Sunflower seeds
- Pumpkin seeds
- Beans
- Soybeans
- Poultry
- Oysters
- Brewer's yeast
- Seafood
- Meats

- Turkey
- Mushrooms
- Wheat germ
- Fortified cereals

Vitamins C and A

Berries and citrus fruits are known for their high vitamin C contents. These are better sources of infection-busting, immune-boosting vitamin C than any supplement. These also do not cause any discomforts like most supplements that contain vitamin C, such as increased gastric acidity. Great natural sources of vitamin A include most yellow and orange-colored vegetables and fruits. This includes carrots, mango, cantaloupe and sweet potato. Both vitamin C and A work together to fight infections and boost immunity. Aside from these, vitamin A and C play vital roles in the development of the cell structure, which is crucial for your baby's growth and development. These vitamins also help in preventing placenta abruption, or the premature separation of the placenta from the lining of the uterus.

DHA

DHA is docosahexaenoic acid. According to the ACOG, pregnant and breastfeeding women should take a minimum of 200 mg per day. This is a great nutrient that improves brain development in babies.

Other Vitamins and Minerals

The following vitamins and minerals are just as essential for a healthy pregnancy and a healthy baby:

Vitamin A and Beta Carotene

- Recommended daily intake: 770 mcg
- Reason for taking: Supports bone growth and teeth development
- Present in these foods:
  - Milk
  - Liver
  - Eggs
  - Cantaloupe
  - Potatoes
  - Broccoli
  - Spinach
  - Carrots
  - Pumpkin
  - Green and yellow vegetables
  - Yellow fruits

Vitamin D

- Recommended daily intake: 5 mcg
- Reasons for taking: aids in the absorption and use of phosphorus and calcium; promotes the development of strong bones and teeth
- Present in these foods:
  - Fatty fish
  - Milk

- ◦ Sunlight exposure

Vitamin E

- Recommended daily intake: 15 mcg
- Reasons for taking: aids in the development of red blood cells and muscles
- Present in these foods:
  - ◦ Spinach
  - ◦ Nuts
  - ◦ Vegetable oil
  - ◦ Fortified cereals
  - ◦ Wheat germ

Vitamin C

- Recommended daily intake: 80 to 85 mcg
- Reasons for taking: antioxidant protecting the tissues from free radical damage; boost immunity; promotes better absorption of iron
- Present in these foods:
  - ◦ Bell peppers
  - ◦ Citrus fruits
  - ◦ Tomatoes
  - ◦ Strawberries
  - ◦ Potatoes
  - ◦ Broccoli
  - ◦ Green beans
  - ◦ Papaya

Vitamin B1 (Thiamine)

- Recommended daily intake: 1.4 mg
- Reasons for taking: increases energy levels; regulates the

growth and development of the nervous system
- Present in these foods:
    - Berries
    - Legumes
    - Nuts
    - Pork
    - Berries
    - Eggs
    - Organ meats
    - Pasta
    - Rice
    - Whole grain
    - Wheat germ
    - Fortified cereals

Vitamin B12 (Riboflavin)

- Recommended daily intake: 1.4 mg
- Reasons for taking: maintains the body's energy levels; promotes healthy skin and good eyesight
- Present in these foods:
    - Fish
    - Poultry
    - Meats
    - Dairy products
    - Eggs
    - Fortified cereals

Vitamin B3 (Niacin)

- Recommended daily intake: 18 mg
- Reasons for taking: promotes better digestion; promotes healthy nerves and skin

30

- Present in these foods:
  - Meats
  - High protein foods
  - Peanuts
  - Milk
  - Fish
  - Eggs
  - Fortified breads and cereals

Vitamin B6 (Pyridoxine)

- Recommended daily intake: 1.9 mg
- Reasons for taking: helps relieve morning sickness; aids in the formation of RBC
- Present in these foods:

  - Liver
  - Chicken
  - Pork
  - Fish
  - Eggs
  - Cantaloupe
  - Bananas
  - Sunflower seeds
  - Walnuts
  - Soybeans
  - Beans
  - Bran
  - Oats
  - Brown rice
  - Wheat germ
  - Cabbage
  - Carrots

- ◦ Spinach
- ◦ Broccoli
- ◦ Beans

Reminders

Again, the source of vitamins and minerals matter just as well as the right amount. There are so many supplements out there that promise to deliver high amounts of any particular mineral or vitamin. One pill can deliver enough vitamins and minerals for the day.

But, while these do contain concentrated amounts of needed minerals and vitamins, supplements are not advisable for pregnant women. Anything artificial is deemed potentially unsafe for the baby. For one thing, there are no studies made on anything artificial with regards to its effects on fetuses, newborns, babies and very young children.

The safest way to go is to go as natural as possible. Another thing is that the body responds better to natural compounds than artificial ones. The body- yours and the baby's- is intrinsically designed to recognize and use natural compounds better. There is an inherent familiarity that results in efficiency and better assimilation. And, naturally occurring minerals and vitamins have much better quality over any of the top artificial, commercial supplements.

Always consult your doctor before you take anything that has been manufactured. This includes supplements, vitamin tablets, mineral supplements and the like. Again, obtain minerals and vitamins from whole, natural sources as much as possible.

Foods You Should Only Eat in Moderation During Pregnancy

Caffeine

There are varying opinions regarding caffeine intake during pregnancy and while breastfeeding. The safest way is this: If not a regular coffee drinker, do not drink during and after pregnancy. If a coffee drinker prior to pregnancy, limit the intake. High amounts of caffeine can have negative effects on the baby's growth and development.

Caffeine is found in coffee, tea and caffeinated versions of certain sodas. Limit intake to not more than any of the following per day (but not all):

- 2 5-oz cups of coffee
- 3 5-oz cups of tea
- 2 12-oz caffeinated soda

In some, babies who have been exposed to high levels of caffeine while they were in their mothers' womb had lower birth weight. Low birth weights tend to increase a baby's risk for certain health problems as he grows older.

Avoid getting more than 200 mg per day. Here is a list of common caffeine-containing compounds and their approximate caffeine contents.

- 1 mug filter coffee: 140mg
- 1 mug instant coffee: 100mg
- 1 can cola: 40mg

- 1 mug tea: 75mg
- 1 can energy drink: 80mg
- 1 50g bar plain (dark) chocolate: less than 25mg (check labels for specific contents)
- 1 50g bar of milk chocolate: less than 10mg

Salty Foods

Limit your salt intake during pregnancy if you don't want to be bloated and edematous. Salt in the blood will attract water, causing an unnecessary rise in blood volume and blood pressure. If too much salt or fluid builds up, serious problems can happen such as edema, cardiovascular complications, and eclampsia.

Preserved, Cured, Processed Meats

You would want to avoid contracting *Listeria* while you are pregnant. During pregnancy, the hormonal changes and the rest of the bodily changes that happen to you lowers your resistance against infection. You will notice it's easier for you to catch a cold. Again, infections-even the simplest ones- are not good for you and your baby.

Your lowered resistance against infection places you at a higher risk for *Listeria*. This is a practically very uncommon infection commonly obtained from eating processed meats like hot dogs. But because of the lowered immunity in pregnancy, you would not want to place yourself and your baby to a higher risk. So best to avoid these:

- Luncheon meats
- Hot dogs
- Cold cuts
- Bologna and other deli meats
- Sausages (dry or fermented)

If you really want to eat, make sure these are heated through and the internal temperatures reach at least 165°F. When served to you, these should be steaming hot to reduce your risk for *Listeria* infection.

When preparing and cooking these meats, avoid getting their juices on any other food. Avoid contact of the liquids from their packages on utensils, other foods and surfaces used for food preparation as well. These liquids from the packaging may contain the infective organism, too.

Pate

Part of food safety during this special time in your life is to avoid refrigerated met spreads or pate from meat counters, deli or refrigerated section of the supermarket. You are not sure if the pate or meat spread did not spend too much time out of refrigeration. If these have been out of cold storage for a prolonged period, microorganisms may have had a chance to colonize and multiply in these foods. Canned meat spreads and pate are safer alternatives than the refrigerated versions. Once the can is opened, transfer to a glass container and store in the refrigerator right after opening.

Foods You Should Only Eat in Small

Amounts While Pregnant

These following foods have been previously thought dangerous but latest studies showed that it does not cause enough damage:

Cheeses

Most soft cheeses may not have been pasteurized. It's best to stay away from cheese traditionally made with unpasteurized milk such as Camembert, queso panela, feta, queso fresco, queso blanco and brie. You can, though, if they are specifically labeled as "made with pasteurized milk".

- *Cheeses that should be avoided during pregnancy include:*

  ◦ Most Soft Cheeses

  ◦ Soft cheese that have white rinds and the soft blue cheese.

  ◦ Soft cheeses have more moisture in side compared to hard cheese. This moisture-rich environment is a great place for bacteria and other infective organisms to multiply. These microorganisms do not commonly cause any problems in humans.

However, because pregnancy changes the body, such as lowering the immune system, a pregnant woman has a higher risk of developing problems with these organisms. Also, these molds have not been tested on fetuses and newborns, so the effects are not predictable.

- These white rinds are molds used to ripen the cheese. Examples include Camembert and brie. It also includes Chevre and other soft goat's cheese that have been ripened with mold. These cheeses may only be eaten if cooked well before eating.

- Soft Blue Cheeses

- Blue-veined soft cheese like Gorgonzola, Roquefort and Danish blue should be avoided. The molds, again, are the issue. These may cause infections, as a pregnant mother generally has a lower immune function. Cook well before using.

- **Safe cheeses to eat include:**

  - All hard cheeses

This includes Stilton, Parmesan and cheddar. Hard cheese can be eaten even without cooking or even if they were made from unpasteurized milk. There is very little moisture in these cheeses compared to soft cheese. This low moisture environment is not hospitable to microbial growth.

  - Mold-ripened soft cheese made with pasteurized milk (check labels):
  - mozzarella
  - cottage cheese
  - feta
  - ricotta
  - cream cheese
  - paneer

- goats' cheese
- halloumi
- processed cheeses, such as cheese spreads

Fresh Vegetables

There was a time when fresh vegetables were discouraged because of the risk for infections like *E. coli* and *Salmonella*. Cooking can kill these infective microorganisms. But sadly, most of the nutrients are also destroyed. But now, experts have given a go for fresh vegetables because of the important nutrients they contain.

Just apply basic food safety such as washing them thoroughly before eating. Wash even if they are brought already bagged and labeled "triple washed." Fruits and vegetables must be washed even if you won't be eating the skin. If not, then any bacteria on the skin will be dragged across the surface of the flesh as you skin them.

Foods Pregnant Women Should Avoid Completely

Getting the right nutrition is not just about eating the right things. It is also about avoiding certain foods that won't do you or your baby any good.

Here are the foods that you should avoid at all costs while you are pregnant.

Processed foods

Junk foods are never good for the body, whether you are pregnant or not. These contain artificial ingredients that can interfere with your baby's growth and development. These artificial compounds also do not promote a healthier body that you need, especially at this point in your life.

Alcohol

In no amount is alcohol safe for the baby. Never take even a small sip of any alcoholic beverage when planning to get pregnant, when you're pregnant and after you give birth. If you are breastfeeding, not a sip, either.

Drinking alcohol is linked to premature delivery and low birth weights. Babies exposed to alcohol while they are still inside their mother's womb have a very high risk of getting FAS or Fetal Alcohol Syndrome.

Rare, raw, under-cooked foods

Food-borne illnesses like *Listeria* are likely to be obtained from foods that have not been cooked thoroughly. Examples include:

- Sushi
- Rare steak
- Under-cooked poultry and meats
- Raw eggs and foods made with raw eggs
- Mayonnaise
- Caesar dressings

Fish

Fish is a healthy source of lean protein, beneficial omega-3 fats and a variety of vitamins and minerals. However, be very cautious on what type of fish you eat. Some fish are known to live in waters that have high mercury levels, methyl mercury or PCB (polychlorinated biphenyls) content. These fish have high possibilities of containing mercury. This heavy metal is an environmental pollutant and has some severe negative effects on the development of your unborn child. It has been known to cause brain damage and developmental delays.

Avoid these fish that are highly likely to have been exposed to polluted or mercury -tainted waters include:

- Tile fish
- Swordfish
- Shark
- King mackerel
- Fish that have high probabilities of getting tainted with PCBs include:
- Bass
- Bluefish
- Trout
- Walleyes
- Freshwater salmon
- Pike

Avoid all fish served seared or raw such as sashimi and sushi. Under-cooked fin-fish is also unsafe. You also would have to pass up under-cooked shellfish like mussels, scallops, clams and oysters.

Eat only 1 type of fish deemed safe each week. Women in their childbearing age should avoid these fish totally even if they are not currently pregnant. The body can store mercury for up to 4 years, and the stored mercury can still affect the baby during this time period.

Eggs

Raw eggs are major sources of *Salmonella* infection. This is a serious infection, especially for pregnant women. Symptoms include diarrhea and vomiting, which can lead to dehydration. It also causes fever and getting a fever during pregnancy isn't a good situation for you or your baby.

Avoid all foods made with raw eggs. Stay away from Caesar salad dressings made in restaurants (which use fresh raw eggs), home made eggnogs, sunny side-up eggs (with a runny yolk), soft scrambled eggs and soft cookie dough. Here is a list of other foods that usually contain raw eggs and must be avoided include:

- Custard
- Ice cream
- Chocolate mousse
- Béarnaise sauce
- Hollandaise sauce

Eggs can still be eaten during pregnancy. They are rich in proteins and fats that can be very beneficial for your baby's growth and development. Just make sure that the eggs are cooked well to remove the risk for *Salmonella* infection.

Sushi

First, check the fish if it's not likely to have exposed to mercury or PCB. Then, check that the fish is thoroughly cooked. Examples are California rolls. Eating uncooked fish in sushi is increasing your risk not just for toxins like mercury, but for parasitic infections as well. If you get sick, you are exposing your baby to the same infection. Also, you would have to choose between riding out the infection until you give birth or risk exposing your child to the toxic effects of antibiotics and other anti-infectives.

You can enjoy eating a maximum of 12 ounces of safe fish per week. This is roughly equivalent to 2 meals. Safe fish, according the latest FDA guidelines, include:

- Canned light tuna
- Shrimp
- Pollack
- Catfish
- Salmon

Make sure these are properly cooked, with internal temperatures of not less than 145°F or until the center turns an opaque color.

For tuna, follow these restrictions because the safety of tuna fish, in terms of mercury-free, cannot be adequately guaranteed. Most people will not experience any mercury toxicity.

However, eating too many tuna during pregnancy may put the baby at risk for mercury exposure.

- Not eating more than 2 tuna steaks (approximately 140 grams when cooked or 170g when raw) per week. OR,
- 4 pieces of medium-sized cans (approximately 140 g each can when drained) of tuna per week

Some fish has abundant healthy fats such as omega-3 fatty acids. However, these omega-3-rich fish are also those that are likely to have been exposed to PCBs and dioxins. Limit consumption of these fatty fish do not more than 2 servings per week. This includes herring, mackerel, trout and salmon.

Smoked fish is generally considered safe to eat during pregnancy. So it's okay to add some smoked trout or smoked salmon to your diet.

Food Rules All Pregnant Women Should Follow

- Always use a food thermometer when cooking meats. The internal temperature is an indicator that the meat has reached temperatures that's considered safe for eating. For lamb, veal and beef, the internal temperatures should reach 145°F.

- For pork and ground meats, the internal temperature must reach 160°F. Poultry should also reach internal temperatures of 165°F. Dishes that contain eggs must reach internal temperatures of 160°F.

- Eggs should be cooked until firm. If the recipe calls for raw eggs, substitute with pasteurized egg products.

- Avoid eating prepared salads in delis, especially those that contain ham, seafood, chicken and eggs. These tend to be sitting around for a long time and microorganisms would have had opportunities to multiply in these.

- Avoid eating foods in picnics or buffets that have been sitting for more than 2 hours.

- Avoid eating stuffing that was cooked inside birds, unless you make sure that the stuffing is heated and reached 165°F.

- Never eat fresh, raw produce that you haven't washed yourself or haven't witnessed someone else wash it, most especially cabbage and lettuce. These have been linked to higher incidence of *Salmonella* cases.

- Leftovers must be heated to 165°F or steaming hot before eating.

- Avoid drinking unpasteurized juices (freshly squeezed), especially if you did not make them yourself. The fruits and/vegetables used might not have been properly washed. The microorganisms on the peel/skin may contaminate the juice.

- Do not eat liver and food that contains liver. This organ meat is high in vitamin A that may not be good for the baby. Examples include liver sausages, haggis, and liver pate.

- Avoid second helpings. This can add too many calories, which will only add to your weight but won't necessarily improve nutrition.

- Limit eating high calorie drinks, snacks and sweets. Your body will not use it for anything. It will only get stored as fat, adding to the postnatal weight you would want to lose.

- When cooking meats or vegetables, choose low-fat, healthy methods. This includes steaming, blanching, baking and grilling.

- Instead of eating 3 large meals per day plus snacks, eat smaller and more frequent meals. Eat 5 to6 small meals a day, then some light snacks in between. This way, you prevent getting too low of levels of blood sugar. This also helps in keeping your energy up all day.

Prenatal Vitamins to Fill the Gaps

Prenatal vitamins are different from other vitamins in many ways. First, they contain more folic acid than the standard multivitamin, as well as more iron. These two elements are extremely important to a pregnant mother and a growing fetus for the following reasons:

- Folic acid helps your baby's brain and spinal cord develop. It can also prevent serious abnormalities of both. Common folic acid deficiency abnormalities can leave your baby seriously handicapped or paralyzed.

- Iron helps your baby to grow and develop. It also prevents mom and baby from becoming anemic, which means that they do not have enough red blood cells in their body.

Prenatal vitamins can also help prevent your baby from being too small for his gestational age, which can be dangerous at birth, AND cause them health problems later in life.

Should You Take Other Vitamins with Them?

All prenatal vitamins are different. Because of this, not all prenatal vitamins contain omega-3, a necessary fatty acid that helps your baby's brain and eyes develop.
If you do not eat fish on a regular basis, or other foods that are high in omega-3 fatty acids, your doctor may recommend a supplement to go along with your prenatal vitamin.

During your second and third trimester, when your baby is growing faster and faster by the day, and his bones are developing at the speed of light, you may need additional calcium and vitamin D supplements.

Depending on your nutritional needs, and the health of your baby, your doctor may recommend that you take a higher dose of folic acid on a regular basis. He will let you know how much more you will need.

Which Prenatal Vitamin is Best?

Even though prenatal vitamins are available over the counter, it is best to get a prescription from your doctor. Not all prenatal vitamins are equal and prescription vitamins contain higher amounts of vitamins.

If you must purchase your prenatal vitamins over the counter, look for a vitamin that is high in vitamin D, vitamin C, vitamin A, vitamin E, zinc, copper and iron.

Prenatal vitamins are not a substitute for a well-rounded, healthy diet. The best thing you can do for your baby is to ensure that you are getting good nutrition daily. Even though these vitamins contain a healthy dose of almost every vitamin you need, they are no where near 100% of the vitamins and minerals you need on a daily basis.

The Ideal Time to Start Taking Prenatal Vitamins

You should begin taking prenatal vitamins as soon as you find out you are pregnant. If your pregnancy is planned, you should begin taking the vitamins as soon as you start trying to become pregnant.

The baby's neural tube, which eventually becomes the baby's brain and spinal cord begins developing during the first month of pregnancy. Typically, a woman is not even aware that she is pregnant during this time.

Breastfeeding moms should continue taking prenatal vitamins until their baby is weaned, in order to supplement baby's diet.

Side Effects of Prenatal Vitamins

There are many women who notice that their prenatal vitamins cause a small bit of nausea. If you are one of the women that feel this side effect, you can remedy this by taking it along with a snack. You can also help to relieve this symptom by taking it before going to bed at night, where the feeling won't bother you as much.

Other side effects that are commonly reported surround constipation. There are many ways to counteract the effect of constipation including:

- Drinking plenty of fluids
- Eating bran flakes in the morning
- Increasing your overall fiber intake
- Become more active physically
- Ask your doctor about stool softeners that are safe to take during pregnancy

If you have tried all of the listed recommendations here, you should consult with your doctor to see if there is a prenatal vitamin that would be easier on your body.

Chapter 4: Exercise During Pregnancy

Accompanying food is exercise. Don't groan – you must keep yourself shape, if only because giving birth can be extremely hard on your muscles! A good exercise regimen can give you strength and endurance enough to help you through not only labor itself, but also the extra weight you'll be carrying during pregnancy as well as body aches like swollen feet or sluggish legs. Also remember, the endorphins released during exercise reduce your stress levels, keeping both you and your baby happy and healthy.

Exercising While Pregnant

Of course, exercising while pregnant is a very delicate process – you *cannot* overdo it under any circumstance, or you risk hurting your baby. Don't let yourself get overheated or dehydrated and practice simple exercises like going for a daily walk. Most experts recommend taking up prenatal yoga, which helps ease labor and delivery. The yoga makes special note of the physical challenges you will face during your pregnancy, like lower back pain, and address those concerns by strengthening your legs, back, abdominal muscles – all muscles essential to delivering a child. The modified moves in prenatal yoga are safe, comforting and soothing; the gentle breathing techniques also act as a great stress reducer.

Once again, keep in mind that before you go in for any kind of exercise program, you should consult your doctor or an experienced friend. Each pregnancy is different and unique;

you will need to find something that is tailored to suit your needs. Keep your caregiver in the loop constantly!

What Exercises Are Safe During Pregnancy?

There are a lot of exercises that can be performed safely during your pregnancy. You just need to be cautious that you don't over exert yourself.

The best exercises are low impact exercises such as brisk walks, swimming, stationary cycling, elliptical machines and aerobics. All of these are activities that can be continues through the pregnancy until birth and are low risk.

There are some activities that are safe for a while, such as racquetball and tennis. Although as you get farther along the fast movements can start to throw you off balance. Jogging is another activity that can be good in moderation. Choosing exercises that do not require a large amount of coordination and balance are best especially when you are farther along.

What Exercises Should You Avoid During Pregnancy?

There are also some exercises that can be dangerous to perform while you are pregnant.

- You should not hold your breath while exercising.
- Any activity that there is a possibility of you falling should not be performed.
- You should not perform any exercise that causes you to jar your mid abdominal area or move quickly changing your direction.

- You should not do activities that include hopping, jumping, bouncing, skipping or running. Sit-ups, knee bends, straight-leg toe touches and leg raises.
- You should not bounce at all while stretching.
- When you stand you should not do activities that require you to twist at the waist.
- You should avoid long periods of inactivity with spurts of heavy exercise.

What Should a Pregnancy Exercise Program Consist of?

As you get farther along in your pregnancy you will notice the changes that are taking place with your body. You should change your activity along with the changes your body makes.

- You and your baby will need more oxygen the farther along you get into your pregnancy
- As pregnancy goes on your body will release hormones that will allow your ligaments to start stretching. This will increase your risk of injury when exercising.
- As you get farther along in your pregnancy your weight will begin to shift from your center of gravity. This added weight will also put more stress on your joints and muscles that are in your lower back and pelvic sections. This will increase your chance to throw off your balance.

What Pregnancy Changes Can Effect Exercise?

You should always take five minutes to wake up and stretch. You can than take fifteen minutes to include cardiovascular activities. When you reach the peak of your activity you should

51

measure your heart rate. Follow this by taking five to ten minutes to gradually slow exercise and end with stretching your muscles gently.

1. You should wear comfortable loose clothing with a comfortable support bra.
2. Having the correct shoes will help to keep you from injuring yourself.
3. You should always exercise on a flat surface.
4. Make sure that if you are exercising that you consume 300 calories more than you already consumes each day.
5. When you eat make sure you finish an hour or more before you exercise.
6. You should always drink water before, in-between and after working out.
7. When you do exercises on the floor you should slowly get to your feet to help prevent yourself from getting dizzy.
8. You should most definitely never over exert yourself during exercise.

Who Should Not Exercise During Pregnancy?

As you get farther along in your pregnancy you will notice the changes that are taking place with your body. You should change your activity along with the changes your body makes.

- You and your baby will need more oxygen the farther along you get into your pregnancy

- As pregnancy goes on your body will release hormones that will allow your ligaments to start stretching. This will increase your risk of injury when exercising.

- As you get farther along in your pregnancy your weight will begin to shift from your center of gravity. This added weight will also put more stress on your joints and muscles that are in your lower back and pelvic sections. This will increase your chance to throw off your balance.

Exercise Warning for Pregnant Women

If you experience any of these symptoms you should stop exercise immediately.

- Have abdominal pain, pelvic pain, or persistent contractions
- Feel chest pain.
- Notice an absence or decrease in fetal movement.
- Have a headache.
- Feel fain, dizzy, nauseous, or light-headed.
- Notice an absence or decrease in fetal movement.
- Have vaginal bleeding.
- Feel cold or clammy.
- Notice an irregular or rapid heartbeat.
- Have a sudden gush of fluid from the vagina or a trickle of fluid that leaks steadily.
- Are short of breath.
- Have sudden swelling in your ankles, hands, face, or calf pain.
- Have muscle weakness.
- Have difficulty walking

Chapter 5: Your Pregnancy by Trimester

Every trimester of your pregnancy will come with its own excitements and challengers. Here, I will break down each trimester and what you can expect as you go.

Three Trimesters

There are three trimesters in your pregnancy that stretch over a span of 40 weeks. Each one brings different symptoms, experiences, excitements, and fears. Here is what you can expect as your pregnancy progresses.

First Trimester

The first three months of your pregnancy are arguably the most difficult and delicate time of your life. Your body begins to change drastically and while we do romanticize the *'pregnancy glow'*, you may also find yourself going through mood swings and irritability, given the various hormonal changes that are happening inside you. Remember, pregnancy is calculated from the last period you had, even though you may have conceived a week or two after it; the first four weeks, you won't even notice a symptom except for the fact that your period did not come as scheduled – this is how you find out that you're pregnant.

Keep in mind; the first three months are when your baby's cells begin to multiply rapidly. You must be extremely cautious and careful during this period – if there is any bleeding or aching, contact your doctor immediately. Exhaustion and morning sickness are normal during this time; so do not get stressed out if you start throwing up at the smell of coffee!

Handling this nausea – morning sickness – can be quite tough. Technically, it is not even *morning* sickness; not every woman throws up in the morning, though a majority report that they start out in the morning sick and the symptoms ease up over the course of the day. The intensity of the sickness also varies from woman to woman; some report constant nausea throughout the day, while others say that they barely felt any sickness at all. There is no hard and fast rule that you will be this sick at this time; you may feel just nauseous, or you may actually throw up. Don't get stressed out about it – just go with the flow and listen to your body!

Typically, morning sickness begins at 6 weeks of pregnancy, though it can start as early as 4 weeks in. it gets worse over the next couple of months – a few women have reported it easing up by the time they hit their 14th week, though it generally lasts till the 18-19th week. It may come and go through the entire duration of your pregnancy, so again, don't expect an exact time frame!

Dealing with morning sickness can be quite painful; regular bouts of nausea and puking are *not* fun, no matter how much we romanticize the beauty of pregnancy. Keeping food down becomes a problem, which means that you may not get the amount of nutrients that you need.

Consult your doctor and see if you can the necessary pills; you want to make sure you remain healthy and keep your baby healthy too. But here are a few quick things you can do to reduce nausea and get some relief from it:

- Eat small and frequent meals through the day so that you're never fully empty; some studies show that protein foods ease the symptoms of nausea.

- Don't lie down immediately after you eat, since that will slow down your digestion.

- Ginger settles your stomach; drink ginger ale, ginger tea and the like to keep your nausea at bay. A good substitute for ginger is peppermint; sucking peppermint candies after eating can also reduce the feeling of wanting to throw up.

- Simple snacks like crackers can ease nausea; keep them by your bedside and munch on them if you wake up in the middle of the night, feeling nauseous.

- Don't jump straight out of bed when you wake up; sit up slowly and spend a couple of minutes breathing in and out deeply.

- Sometimes, strong smells can trigger the feeling of nausea. Avoid these; eat food at room temperature or cold – hot food has stronger aroma that can make you feel like throwing up.

- Drink fluids, particularly sour drinks like lemonade, between meals.

- Add sports drinks with glucose, salt, potassium and the like to replace any lost electrolytes from too much vomiting.

- Get fresh air. A stuffy room is nauseating even to non-pregnant people; it adds to your distress when you're carrying a baby.

- Stress also adds to nausea, so spend time relaxing and unwinding.

- Use aromatherapy; some women have reported that some smells keep the nausea at bay while others trigger it. Smells of lemon, mint and orange have generally been accepted as settling the stomach, so buy a fresh lemon and keep it by your bedside when you feel too sick.

If your nausea is not abating in the least and becomes more than you can handle, you may have to consult your doctor. You could be suffering from other conditions like *hyperemesis gravidarum*; in which case, your doctor will want to provide you with special treatment. Talk to your OB-GYN regularly and keep them updated so that they can help you at all times!

Second Trimester

In contrast to the first trimester, the second is almost a breeze through. For most women, the nausea abates, leaving them able to enjoy the pregnancy and *'glow'*. By the fourth month, your belly starts rounding out, showing the outward sign of your pregnancy. By the time you hit 20 weeks, you should be able to feel your baby's movements, starting out as small flutters, which will gradually progress to out and out kicks and jabs as you come closer to your due date.

During this time, make sure you eat a lot of fruits and

vegetables. Also make sure you drink a lot of water to keep constipation away. *Enjoy* your pregnancy; don't worry too much about the changes your body is undergoing. A lot of women go through insecurities regarding their appearance, particularly about your weight. This is normal; don't get too stressed out about it!

Make sure you get enough sleep. With the baby moving around inside you at odd hours of the night, you may not be able to get a full night's rest as you need. In that case, add a 30-60 minute nap to your routine. This will make you more alert, sharpen your memory and reduce any fatigue you may experience. Remember though, nap for too long and you run the risk of not being able to sleep at night!
Exercising can also help you get to sleep better. It will leave you tired, so you fall into deep slumber as soon as you hit the bed. But space it out properly; exercise revs you up and makes you more energetic immediately after you've completed it, so allow 3-4 hours in between your work out and your bedtime so that you're just the right amount of fatigued to sleep comfortably.

Also train yourself to sleep on your sides. Lying on your side helps the blood flow and ensures that your baby is receiving all nutrients it needs; most women report that it is the most comfortable position to sleep in when their bellies become bigger.

Third Trimester

These are the last few months of your pregnancy. Your body will feel huge and heavy, and you may feel heartburn often. Some women even report being unable to take large meals and being breathless often. Your baby's movements will, however, become restricted, given that there is very little room for him/her to move around now.

This is the crucial time when you need to be on constant watch. You could go into labor at anytime, particularly if you're carrying twins – rarely do multiple pregnancies come to full term. Some women may experience false contractions or what is known as Braxton Hicks, as you edge closer to your delivery date – they're nothing to be worried about. It's just your uterus getting ready to deliver the baby.

However, since it can be difficult to differentiate between real contractions and Braxton Hicks, you should be very cautious and contact your doctor immediately if you feel them; you don't want to take any risk with your baby's health! One way to distinguish between real contractions and Braxton Hicks is to exercise – the former is strong enough that you will be able to feel them even when you're working out. The false contractions, on the other hand, are slight enough that you may or may not notice them while exercising. In either case, contact your doctor right away and get the prognosis confirmed.

Once again, eat healthy, get enough rest and practice your prenatal yoga. As you are entering into your third trimester, start getting things ready for the actual birth. By now, you should have completed baby proofing your house and getting all the other practical side of things done. If not, get started right away! Here is a quick checklist of things you are going to have to get done –

9. Baby proof your house of all choking hazards

10. Get the nursery ready

11. Buy/assemble a crib for your baby; get a baby

monitor

12. Have baby clothes, shoes and the like ready

13. Make sure you have bucket loads of diapers ready – *you will need it!*

Of course, these are the most basic things you should get done in anticipation of your child's arrival. Sort things out at your work to see how long you can take off; find a good sitter or a day-care center that will look after your newborn when you return to work. It may seem like you're rushing with these decisions, and you may ask why get all this done so early when your baby hasn't even been *born* yet – believe me, you won't have a minute to yourself once your bundle of joy arrives! Get all these chores out of the way so that you can focus on taking care of your baby and recuperating after you give birth.

This is also the time when you will need to decide what you are going in for – a home birth or checking into a hospital. While most women prefer to opt for the latter, a few may choose to give birth at home, where they are most comfortable and therefore, are less likely to be stressed about. In any case, the choice is yours – just keep your OB-GYN up to date and ensure that they're on board with whatever you want. Of course, there may be complications in your case, meaning that you may not have a choice. Whatever you decide, make sure it is the best possible option for both you and your child.

In case you are going to the hospital, make sure you have a labor bag packed well in advance. As you know, you cannot predict exactly when you'll go into labor, so make sure you have everything you will need gathered and ready to go at a moment's notice!

With all that done, you are officially ready to give birth!

Chapter 6: Labor

The actual labor process itself is one that is painful – there is *no* other word for it. You're going to be pushing a human being out of your vagina; it's certainly not a joke to be taken lightly! Active labor can last up to 8 hours, with another hour or two of pushing to get your baby out. Of course, this is once again an average number; first time mothers generally report undergoing longer hours of labor, though it's never more than 20-24 hours.

To give you a short gist of what happens in your body when you go into active labor – you will be in a latent phase of labor through the last weeks of your pregnancy. This is when you will experience Braxton Hicks – if you do – as your uterus prepares to deliver. In active labor, your cervix begins to dilate and the baby – typically the baby's head – begins to descend down to your vagina. Needless to say, the dilation process is painful. When the cervix is fully dilated to 10cm, your doctor will instruct you to push and you can birth your child. Following the baby's birth is the cutting of the umbilical cord that ties the baby to you. The doctor will clamp and then cut the cord, after which the baby will be cleaned and handed to you.

You could also opt for a water birth. This may sound frightening, but many women have reported that getting into water when they're in labor and giving birth in water reduces the labor pain to a vast extent. They claim that the water allows for a more comfortable position and acts as a sedative. Immersing themselves in the soft liquid reduces stress and anxiety related hormones.

However, do keep in mind that medically, water births have not been proven to make much of a difference; in fact, one will have to be exceptionally careful with the baby coming out to make sure it doesn't drown. Critics are still arguing the benefits and the adverse effects and studies are still going on to develop it further. If you do choose to go in for this, make sure you have experts on your side! Discuss it with your doctor/midwife and choose the best option available to you.

Of course, these are natural births, which is what most doctors' aim for. In case of complications or emergencies, your OB-GYN will decide to prep you for a C-Section or a cesarean birth, in which case, the baby will be surgically removed from your uterus. Don't worry about that – trust your doctor to know what to do!

Remember, to reduce pain during labor, you could go in for epidural shots. But some women choose to go the natural way without any pain medication. It's your choice – discuss it openly and honestly with your doctor and then make a rational decision.

Packing for the Hospital

Now, for those women who have chosen to go to the hospital for labor, you will need to pack a labor bag! We already discussed this in the previous chapter; here are a few quick things you need to pack into the bag, listed out by experienced mothers who have been through it all before –

- A bathrobe/nightgown, slippers and socks with a change of clothes; obviously, you don't want to continue wearing hospital scrubs or your messy clothes after you give birth. Choose something loose, preferably sleeveless, so that you can't your blood pressure checked easily. Your slippers and the robe will be helpful if you want to walk outside your room when you're in labor.

- Toiletries for you, since your stay will likely extend for a couple of days – make sure you have your toothbrush, toothpaste, hairbrush, soap and whatever else you require for personal grooming. Some women even take make-up along with them to help them feel confident when they get discharged – pack whatever you think you'll need!

- Nursing bras or comfortable normal bras is something essential; you may or may not choose to breastfeed, but your breasts are likely to be swollen and tender when the milk comes in. A good bra is comfort personified and you can add breast pads to absorb any leaks.

- Add maternity underpants; the hospital-provided mesh underwear may or may not be comfortable for you. Try on different brands before you give birth so that you don't go wrong after labor! Also pack sanitary pads in case you bleed after delivery – it is not an uncommon phenomenon and tampons will be painful in this state, so stick to napkins for now.

- Anything to help you relax, like your own pillow/blanket that will soothe you through the pain.

- For your partner, who will be accompanying you into the delivery room – pack a camera, if you want to record the birth, along with batteries and a memory card. Of course, hospitals may or may not allow filming of the actual birth, but in any case, a few videos after the baby is born is always fun to do!

- A small snack treat after you deliver is a good idea; hospital food is not always the most delicious of fares!

- A bag of diapers for the baby without doubt!

- For the baby, make sure you have an entire outfit packed properly for the day you take him/her home. Socks, booties and a full outfit – bring your bundle of joy home in style! Also add a blanket the hospital will provide a blanket while you're with them, but it may be a good idea to swaddle your sweetheart in the blanket as you take them home as well.

- Make sure your car seat is installed properly so that you can take your newborn home safely.

This is just a quick checklist to get you started. Remember, each pregnancy is different and each person has their own needs, so pack all that you feel you will need. Also keep in mind that you aren't going away on a long holiday – you'll be at the hospital for not more than a week or so. Pack wisely and get it ready well in advance so that you're not running around when you're actually in labor.

Preparing for Childbirth

Now that you are closer to your baby's due date after nine months of eagerness and hope. With the last few months coming along you will start to feel your uterus begin to tighten. These annoying and obnoxious phases of tightening are referred to as Braxton Hicks contractions. The Braxton Hicks contractions warm up the uterus for the trials that are set for it down the road and will make it easier when labor starts.

False labor can be another annoying dilemma that can be annoying when you are close and expecting the real labor to start.

Deciphering Real Labor from False Labor:

For any first time mother a false labor can become very scary. This happens when there are frequent more intense Braxton Hicks contractions. When this happens you should get yourself to the hospital or get a hold of your midwife. This is something that is normal and you will find out when you get to the hospital and you should not find yourself ashamed of it. When you are pregnant it is always better to be safe and not take the risk of holding off and end up delivering in a car instead of at a hospital.

Signs of False Labor

For any first time mother a false labor can become very scary. This happens when there are frequent more intense Braxton Hicks contractions. When this happens you should get yourself to the hospital or get a hold of your midwife. This is something that is normal and you will find out when you get to the hospital and you should not find yourself ashamed of it. When you are pregnant it is always better to be safe and not take the risk of holding off and end up delivering in a car instead of at a hospital.

- If there is no labor progression over time
- Irregular or unpredictable contractions
- If you change positions and contractions stop
- If you only feel generalized contractions
- If there is no bloody or cervical mucus showing evidence of your water breaking.

True Labor

True labor is unlike any experience you will ever feel. Even if you have been through false labor, do not expect true labor to be a similar experience. Here is what you should expect from true labor.

Predicting when labor will start is still not 100% possible even though there is so much technology now of days. When you get a due date from your doctor it is a reference given factoring in when you got pregnant. These are never completely accurate because labor can come as early as 3 weeks before the given date, or up to 2 weeks later. There are some ways your body can show signs that labor will be starting soon.

Signs of Labor

You will begin to have a lighter feeling. This occurs when the baby turns and its head travels to the pelvic area preparing for the birthing process. When this happens you will begin to breathe a little easier because the baby will not be squeezing your lungs. Your belly will also lower. When this happens you will also start to feel like you will need to pee more because your baby will now be pressing on your bladder.

Your mucus plug will release that seals your uterus from any infections. This will cause a brownish discharge that is blood tinged from the cervix.

Labor can also cause bowel movements that are more frequent and loose.

If you have gushing or fluid leaking from your vagina than your amniotic sac membranes have probably burst. These are the membranes that surround your baby and protect it during the pregnancy. If your body does not go into labor naturally within 24 hours your doctor will probably try to avoid delivery infections and complications by stimulating labor.

You will start experiencing periodic contractions irregularly as your labor becomes nearer. When you start having 10 minute intervals of contractions that this could be a sign of labor starting.

Stages of Labor

There are 3 phases to the first stage of labor: Latent, Active and Transition.

Stage 1

The first phase is the longest and least intense phase, known as the latent phase. Your contractions will become more frequent to help your cervix to dilate and help move your baby towards the birth canal. When your cervix begins to thin out dilate and efface you will experience light discomfort. You may be admitted by your doctor to the hospital if your contractions stay regular. This is so that he or she can examine you frequently checking the dilation of your cervix.

When you start into the active phase your cervix will begin to dilate quickly. You will begin to experience a strong pain from pressure in your back or abdomen with every contraction. You will also start to feel like you need to push or bear down on impulse but you will need to wait until your cervix has become dilated completely.

When you hit the Transition stage your cervix will become dilated up to 10 cm. You will now experience strong and painful contractions frequently. These contractions can last 1 to 1.5 minutes and start up about every 3 to 4 minutes.

Stage 2

When your cervix becomes dilated completely you will hit the second stage of your labor. You will now be told to start pushing. Your pushing with the contractions can help to push the baby into the birth canal. The baby can squeeze through the small birth canal because of the baby's soft spots (fontanels) on its head.

Your baby will begin to crown when its head reaches the vaginal opening which is the biggest part. Your doctor will begin to suction amniotic fluid and mucus from the mouth and nose of your baby when its head comes out. You will need to aid in delivering the body and shoulders of your baby by pushing.

Now that you have delivered your baby the doctor will clamp

the umbilical cord and the doctor or your partner will need to be cut.

Stage 3:

Now that your baby has been delivered you are at the final and 3rd stage of labor. The placenta is the organ that fed your baby when he or she was in the uterus. This will now be removed during this stage.

Labor can be different for many women. Since you are a first timer you will probably have a labor and delivery that will last from twelve to fourteen hours. Each time you have a pregnancy you can expect the times of labor to shorten.

Pain Treatments

There are also different pains that can be felt during labor and delivery with different women. Factors such as contraction strength and size or even the position of the baby can influence the pain that you experience. Some women can manage some of the pain that is learned by going to classes for childbirth. They can show you how to relax and how to breathe to help. Medications or other options that are non-drug related may help other women to cope with the pain.

Medications.

There are certain side effects that you can experience from medications given during labor even when they are safe for both you and the baby. You could be given analgesic medications or anesthetics by your doctor.

The anesthetics can block movement, feeling and pain. When you are given general anesthetics you will become unconscious. If you are having a C-section you will be given general anesthesia or an epidural. Depending on your medical facts for you, your pregnancy and your baby it will be determined by your doctor what anesthesia to administer to you.

You will lose all feeling and movement in your muscles along with relieving pain when given analgesics. This can be administered systematically by injections into the muscle, vein or even your back to help anesthetize the lower portion of your body.

They can also relieve pain quickly by conducting a spinal black that is injected once into the spinal fluid. Pain medication can be continuously administered using an epidural block into spinal cord where the region of spinal nerves are located. They do this by a catheter injection into the epidural area. The side effects that can be expected are lower blood pressure, headaches and they can slow down your baby's heart rate.

Non-Drug Alternatives

There are some alternatives that are non-drug related. Changing your position frequently, using techniques to relax, acupuncture and hypnosis can help to relieve pain. Discussing medication options with your doctor to help cope with pain is still a good idea even if you plan on managing pain without them.

After the Delivery

While your body is recovering from the childbirth your body will go through transitions. Here is a list of transitions you will experience physically.

- Your breast and nipples will swell and become painful when they begin to produce milk.

- You will experience a heavier than normal bloody vaginal discharge than your normal menstruation. In the next two months this will fade to a yellow or a white and stop.

- Because your uterus is returning to its original size over the next few days you may continue to experience more contractions. These can occur more often while you are nursing.

- You will most likely feel pain while walking and sitting in the areas where the doctor has performed an episiotomy. This is where the doctor has created a cut between the vagina and anus to allow for an easier birth. This is known as the perineum.

- You may have some uncontrolled bowel movements or urine leaks when you laugh or sneeze. This is because of the extended stress and stretching that occurs during your baby's delivery. As your body heals you will gain more control over these issues.

- During childbirth and pregnancy it is common for varicose veins and the anal to become inflamed causing hemorrhoids.

- As hormonal levels and blood flow stabilizes to adjust after childbirth you will experience hot and cold flashes.

- For the next couple of days following child birth you may experience constipation. Sore muscles, hemorrhoid and episiotomy can also lead to pain when you have a bowel movement.

Baby blues are experienced by about 80 percent of all new mothers. This can cause you to experience constant crying, irritability and sadness for a couple days to weeks after giving birth. These baby blues could be related to the hormonal changes and exhaustion that is experienced with adjustments that need to be made to incorporate your baby into your lifestyle.

If these baby blues continue and do not fade you should consult your doctor. You could be experiencing postpartum depression. This can come about in 10 to 25 percent of all new mothers.

Induction of Labor

Many women hear the topic of induction and they do not know exactly how to respond. The thought that your body does not want to go into labor on its own, or that your baby would be safer if they were delivered under a medical induction can be terrifying. However, if you take the time to understand the process, it will not be nearly as scary as it sounds.

What is Medical Labor Induction?

There are many medical reasons to have your labor induced. Your body naturally creates the hormones necessary to start your labor. However, some women do not create enough of the hormone to really get labor going strong enough to bring your baby into this world. Sometimes, your body just needs a little boost.

When your doctor has decided that it is time to induce your labor, he will give you an IV medication called pitocin. This will help start contractions and help to thin out your cervix.

Who Should Be Considered for Induction?

There are many reasons that your doctor may consider you for induction. These reasons are:

- gestational diabetes
- pre-eclampsia
- going past your due date (41 weeks pregnant)
- if the health of you and your baby are at risk by continuing the pregnancy
- ... and other medical conditions that affect you and baby

What about inducing for non-medical reasons?

Are you just tired of being pregnant? Or does your doctor have something planned during the time of your due date? Does this have you thinking about inducing early? Did you know that almost 25 percent of the inductions are not medically necessary or are elective according to the Center for Disease Control Moms and experts are hot on the topic of induced labor during non-medical reasons.

Inducing before 39 weeks have not been recommended by the American College of Obstetricians and Gynecologists. If you induce earlier than 39 weeks there is a risk of bringing a child into the world that is not fully developed. "Induction can carry risks that should only be used for medical reasons," says Sabine Droste, MD. She is a professor at the University of Wisconsin-Madison of obstetrics and gynecology.

There are certain situations where if the doctor thinks that they are close to deliver but live too far away or won't make the drive to the hospital the doctor may make a call to induce. This would keep a birth from happening on the road, or anywhere outside of the hospital.

What are the risks of non-medical induction?

There are times when family come to see the birth of your child or we are so busy that we would like to have the delivery at a certain time. This can cause for a treat amount of temptation to induce your pregnancy because of this. Other times people think and say that you are too big and you will have to have a C-section in order to have your child. This can scare mothers to try and induce labor before truly knowing if the baby really is too big or not.

You should really think about this and be cautious because you could complicate things. Just because you induce early does not mean you will not need to have a C-section. The chances of having a C-section are about as equal of a chance as the baby actually being too big to need a C-section. You should wait to make this decision after discussing with your doctor the options you have taken and thought about.

How is labor induced?

When there is a patient that has a cervix that is insufficiently dilated, the cervix needs to be softened. We do this by using prostaglandin which is a hormone. After the cervix is softened another hormone called oxytocin is administered to help trigger labor. Pitocin is usually intravenously administered. Inducing labor is much easier when there are already signs of labor early on. This is because the body is ready to go.

There are other ways of inducing labor, such as breaking the amniotic sac releasing the amniotic fluid. This is done by puncturing the amniotic sac with a sterile plastic like hook. When the amniotic fluid is released it contains prostaglandins. This will help to increase the frequency and strength of your contractions. If this does not induce labor than there is a larger risk that infection can spread to your baby because there are no fluids to protect the baby any more.

There is a different procedure called membrane sweeping. This involves breaking the membrane connections from the uterus. This is supposed to force the cervix to start dilating and effacing which should help to start contractions.

Although these are methods that are used, it does not mean that they will always work. It all depends on how the mothers body will react when these actions are taken. The mothers body can react differently to any of these. It could cause labor to run fast and smooth or it could make things take longer.

Do natural induction methods really work?

Here are popular methods that are used. You can decide for yourself if they are effective.

Walking has been used to try and help move the baby into a position that uses gravity that can help.

Stimulating your nipples can help release oxytocin and can start contractions. Although doctors give caution to this method because it can also cause contractions that will last longer and cause distress to your baby.

The Pineapple fruit has a chemical in it called bromelain. This can help to soften the tissues connected to the cervix.

Sex can be a fun way of trying to speed things along. This is because semen has cervix-softening prostaglandins in it.

Spicy foods can also help kick the body into full gear and get your innards moving. But if it does not work it could just cause you to have gas.

Having a C-Section

There are so many women who have their birth plan in mind through their full pregnancy.

They have memorized and read about all the details. Many end up learning that the best chance for the safety of their child is for them to be delivered through C-section. This can be upsetting when this was not the plan they had in mind all this time. This change in plans can cause the feeling of fear, guild and dread causing them to tailspin. In all reality women should always keep in mind that things can and may happen to change how the delivery of their baby may go.

The C-section is no way any woman wants the birth to go but in certain situations it becomes necessary. Here we will discuss what you can expect if your doctor says the better way is to have a C-section. Sometimes the doctor may call that a C-section should be done because of certain complications that the doctor has noticed. Other times it happens during labor when the baby is not reacting well with the contractions you are having.

When a mother hears C-section mentioned it automatically causes fear to develop. We will discuss issues that are common with unplanned C-sections.

Typical Immediate Fears

C-sections are commonly talked about and how they are so awful. This can cause instant dread and questions to flood your mind. Some of these worries are would it ruin my experience of birth? Will there be an excruciating and long recovery time? Would I be left with big ugly scars?

Will this C-section be unnecessary?

The decision in performing a C-section is made by 2 physicians. They are quite common and happen in 1 out of 4 births. Some reasons that C-sections are taken into account are for multiple pregnancy, large baby, labor failure, diabetic medical conditions, fetal distress, placenta Previa or high blood pressure.

Will the Surgery be Long and Scary?

It is normal for any major surgery to make you apprehensive. You will feel pressure and a slight tugging when they pull the baby out. It should be a painless procedure that takes around 45 minutes. The baby is usually born within 10 to 15 minutes from the start of the operation.

Most of the C-section is performed with the mother awake. To relieve pain the mother can have a spinal block or epidural which will numb the lower portion of the body.

Epidurals are usually used in labor and it will be topped off before the surgery of a C-section. The Spinals are given when there is a scheduled cesarean. They last only about 1 or 2 hours and can be easily administered. They reserve general anesthesia in rare cases or emergencies when the spinal or epidural does not work.

The surgery starts with an incision above the bikini line into the abdomen wall. A second incision is made in the uterus wall where the delivery of the baby takes place. They then cut the umbilical cord and remove the placenta and close the incisions.

When the surgery is all done Duramorph is usually administered for a long-lasting pain reliever. This helps for any discomfort after the spinal or epidural has stopped working.

Will this rob me of the experience of giving birth?

It is not a regular birth but the mother is awake and will experience her baby being delivered into this world and into her arms.

You should not blame yourself for a C-section and that the planned labor did not go as was planned. As long as the baby is healthy and delivered than the birth was a success. You should be happy that you just brought a life into this world.

Will a C-section prevent me from bonding with my baby?

When you have a C-section you are awake to witness it and most times you will have your baby handed to you right after birth. This allows for you to hold your baby and love them.

Will recovery be extremely painful and difficult?

You are held for around 4 days at the hospital where you will experience pain around the areas where the incisions were made. It will also be difficult to get out of bed and back in bed unassisted. You will be given a couple of types of drugs to help manage pain. Percocet will most likely be prescribed as a painkiller. Sometimes a morphine drip that can be self-administered will be given so that the patient can press a button when the pain gets to be too much.

There are ways that you can help to lower the pain and increase the speed of recovery. Drinking warm water has been suggested. This can help you to pass gas. This shows that you can start eating solid foods again. It is also suggested that if you have had a C-section that you get out of bed the day after surgery or as soon as possible.

This helps to loosen up the muscles around the incision area and can get you back to wanting to get up and go.

Medication will help to ease the pain so that you can get out of bed and you shouldn't be afraid to use it.

When you get home keep getting up and moving but don't over work yourself and do strenuous work. You will begin to feel better in as little as a week.

Will I have a scary, ugly scar?

At first the area can be red. There will be a thin scar just above your pubic hairline. The incisions are usually 5 to 6 inches in length so that there is enough room for the shoulders and head of your baby to be delivered. Over time the color and size of your scar will face where only your husband, doctor and if you have one your bikini waxer will only see. You can also look at your scar as a happy remembrance of when you brought your child into this world.

Will all of my future babies have to be born through C-section?

Doctors for the longest time always stuck with the saying that once you had a C-section you would always have a C-section. This is no longer how it is looked at. There is now a 70% success rate of vaginal birth after cesarean and it is increasing as a safe option.

But as with any surgery there can always be more complications that can cause serious risk. You should always allow your doctor to consider and evaluate if it is an option for your next birth or not. Always make sure to consult your doctor and ask those important questions in moderation during your office visits.

Chapter 7: Post Natal Care

Now, what films and books tend to do is ignore the discomforts of looking after newborns while your body is still going through changes. They rush straight into the *being a glowing mother* part of things; let me tell you right now that rarely ever happens. Don't have unrealistic expectations of what your life is going to be like once you bring your newborn home – it will be a beautiful and amazing experience, but it will also be difficult and tough, as most good things in life are.

It goes without saying that your attention should be focused on looking after your newborn. We will discuss that in the next chapter. But as important as taking care of your baby is, it's equally essential that you keep an eye on yourself! Vaginal births are often accompanied with other tough body changes that you need to be able to handle; ignoring these problems could lead to major complications later on. From vaginal soreness to urinary problems, you could have a number of difficulties that you will need to handle immediately. Here are a few of these issues –

Vaginal Soreness

If you had a vaginal tear when you delivered, then the wound may take a while to heal and seal closed. Don't worry about it too much about it; these are natural and happen often. However, make sure you sit on a pillow or a comfortable surface so that you don't aggravate your wound.

Make use of a squeeze bottle and pour a little warm water over your vulva when you pee; have a clean pad or wash cloth to hold firmly against the wound when you are pooping. This will soothe the pain and keep it from getting aggravated.

An ice pack is also a good idea, but it may be uncomfortable initially. Take painkillers as ordered by your doctor.

Keep in mind that it will slowly improve as you heal. If the discomfort worsens, and your wound becomes swollen, hot or you see pus-like discharge, contact your doctor immediately to avoid infections and the like.

Vaginal Discharge

For a few weeks after you've delivered your baby, you will have a vaginal discharge. A flow of heavy blood is something you can take for granted for the first few days; you'll have to wear sanitary napkins instead of tampons, since inserting anything into your vagina will no doubt be painful for a while. The discharge will slowly turn colors from red to pink to brown and then to yellow or white. It will turn water and then taper off.

This is nothing to worry about. Only get in touch with your doctor if your bleeding becomes heavier, if the discharge stinks or you contract a fever or 100.4 F or higher.

Contractions

Even after labor and delivery, you may experience contractions. These after-pains resemble your usual monthly menstrual cramps, but they will fade away with time, so ask your doctor to prescribe over-the-counter pain relievers if you find it too painful! If you have a fever, though, these could be indicative of a uterine infection, so get in touch with your doctor immediately.

Urinary Problems

After you give birth, the tissues that surround your bladder or urethra could swell up or get bruised, which means that you will find it hard to pee. The perineal area could also be very tender from birthing the baby, so when you urinate, you could experience a sharp sting or even slight pain. The best thing to do is to pour water across your vulva as you are sitting on the toilet; the difficulty in peeing will solve itself.

Don't panic if you wet your underwear even without needing to pee. Pregnancy and childbirth stretch the connective tissue at the base of the bladder; it can cause damage to the nerves and muscles of the bladder/urethra. You will leak urine in this case, as you cough or laugh or do any excessive movement. Relax – this will solve itself over time! Just wear sanitary pads; speak to your doctor about the kind of exercises you can do to tone up your pelvic muscles.

But if the urge to urinate persists, and/or you continue to feel a burning sensation when you pee, call your doctor. You could be suffering an infection that will require treatment.

Remember, doing *Kegel* exercises will help you. *Kegels* are a set of exercises developed to strengthen your pelvic muscles. Start by tightening those muscles, as if you were trying to stop a stream of urine while peeing. Then let go gently; try it for 5 seconds at a time, 4-5 times at a go. Slowly increase it to keeping your muscles contracted for around 10 seconds. Repeat it 10 times in a day. Again, consult your doctor to make sure you're doing these correctly.

Hemorrhoids and Bowel Movements

Some women may experience pain while they pass stools, or find their anus swollen soon after birth. These are symptoms of hemorrhoids, which is basically a condition where the veins in the anus or lower rectum swell up. Contact your doctor immediately; he/she will give you medications and tell you what to do.

Soaking in a warm tub and applying a chilled witch hazel pad to the swollen area will soothe the pain. To avoid extra pain while passing stools, try to keep your poop soft and regular. Eat foods with a high content of fiber, from fruits and vegetables to whole grains. Drink a lot of water to avoid constipation and if needed, ask your doctor for a laxative to help you poop comfortably.

Another bowel problem for new mothers is the inability to control your bowel movements, which, as you can expect, can be quite uncomfortable and embarrassing. Practice your *Kegel* exercises daily to help with your fecal leakage; if your problem persists, contact your doctor to see what can be done.

Sore and Leaking Breasts

This is not necessarily a problem that has to be worried about, but it is an issue that can be painful for a lot of mothers. Soon after you give birth, your breasts will become swollen, tender and may even be engorged in size. It's possible you already experience something similar during your pregnancy; your body is preparing to feed your baby, whether or not you go the breastfeeding route.

Obviously, it is not the most comfortable of feelings; nursing is the best option to reduce discomfort. Use a breast pump if you can and apply cool, soft wash cloths to soothe any irritability in between feeding your baby.

If you decide not to breastfeed, then wear a firm, supportive bra – like a sports bra – that will help stop the production of milk. If you pump your breast, or rub it, it will only increase the milk production.

Wear nursing pads inside your bra to help with leaking milk between feedings; remember to change these pads as soon as you are done feeding and they are fully soaked.

Hair Loss and Changes in your Skin

When you are pregnant, your hormone levels are elevated. One side effect of this is that your hair becomes thicker, lusher and grows really well. The downside is that when you deliver, your body sheds all this extra hair at a go. For six months, you may experience heavy hair loss – don't worry about it! It's natural. Once your body flushes out the excess hormones and you go back to normal, your hair will also look just fine.

And of course, the terrifying stretch marks will also appear during pregnancy. Don't worry too much about them; apply Shea butter lotion or something similar to keep it under control. They should eventually fade to silver or white color and become barely noticeable. Any skin that went dark during your pregnancy will also turn back to normal.

Mood Swings

The baby blues are not a myth. Yes, motherhood is beautiful and is the most wonderful thing a woman can experience; but it also painful and disturbing. Once the initial giddiness wears off, there is no doubt that you will feel down, depressed and anxious. Couple this with the lack of sleep that comes from taking care of an infant that keeps his/her own hours, and it is no wonder that you go through mood swings! Your hormone levels are still wonky at this point, so if you feel down in the dumps, then there is nothing wrong with it!

Have people around you to help out with your baby. Looking after the infant by yourself will stress you out even more – make your partner take over for a little while and put your feet up. Relax and get enough sleep and allow your body to naturally correct itself over the course of time instead of fretting and fuming.

Of course, if the blues persist and don't leave even after 10-12 days after delivery, you must contact your doctor. You could be suffering from something called 'postpartum depression', which is a common phenomenon many mothers go through, especially for prematurely born babies. Symptoms include:

- Anxiety, restlessness

- Loss of interest in life

- Not feeling hungry

- Problems with your sleep (not related to your child causing lack of sleep)

- Feeling worthless

- Feeling guilty or helpless

- Feeling little interest in the baby

- Sudden weight gain/loss

There is no need to panic; postpartum depression is easily treated. Just contact your doctor if you feel these symptoms and get started on it right away – letting it linger could make it difficult for you to bond with your baby. And as we all know, the initial bonding period between parent and child is very important for the formative years!

Chapter 8: Looking After a Newborn

Bringing home a baby can be terrifying. You have a new human being, entirely dependent on you for every single thing, from being fed to being cleaned. Your child cannot do anything for itself, which means it's fragile and delicate and have to be cared for. It's a daunting prospect, to say the least. But don't panic! As many as your baby's needs are, you are fully capable of meeting them; you've already come far, having carried him/her through nine months of pregnancy and birthed them. Now, you look after them!

Here are a few quick things you must remember when you first receive the baby from the nurse –

- Wash your hands before you touch your baby; he/she still has only a weak immune system and are susceptible to infection.

- Support the baby's head and neck; he/she is so tiny they cannot even hold up their head on their own. Cradle the head whenever you carry your newborn.

- Don't ever shake your newborn, even in play! Vigorous shaking may lead to bleeding in the brain, leading even to death. If you want to wake your baby up, blow gently over a soft cheek or tickle those tiny feet.

- Limit any activity that is rough or bouncy; your baby is still extremely delicate and needs to rest.

Feeding

Feeding your baby for the first time is an extremely satisfying experience. It doesn't matter whether you formula feed, or breastfeed, you will be able to bond with your baby right from the start.

- **Breastfeeding**

The first few times when you feed your newborn, you're going to be anxious and worried since you've never done it before. Don't panic; just hold your baby close to your breast and allow him/her to seek it out and suck.

On the first day, your baby will feed anywhere between 8-15 times, given that the stomach is tiny. For those who are breastfeeding keep practicing latching your baby to your breast – the doctor/midwife should instruct you in this initially, so ask for help if you need it! Try out different positions until you feel comfortable.

Remember to bring your baby to your breast and not the other way around; feed him/her before he starts crying really loudly, because then, the tongue will be too far back in their mouth. Soothe and calm them before you start feeding them and *never* force them onto your breast.

Once they've finished feeding, they will become sleepy and relaxed and come off your breast themselves. Keep him/her raised up on a cushion or a pillow for support; the first feeds tend to take 40 minutes or even longer than that. Be patient, relaxed and enjoy the closeness with your child. Don't worry if they move away within a few minutes; some babies feed for a long time, while others don't. Just make sure they're latched on properly and get all the food they need.

• Bottle Feeding

For those who are bottle-feeding, things get a bit trickier. You may need to take larger amounts of formula milk than a breastfed baby. Make sure he/she is comfortably settled on your lap, with you supporting the head. Tip the bottle and keep it horizontal so that they aren't flooded with milk and aim the teat at the roof of the baby's mouth to get him/her to suck at the nipple.

If your baby slows down or rests when eating, then chances are they've had enough. Pause for a moment to let them decide if they're full; if they start sucking again, then they're not. Then, gently pull the bottle away and hold them up, stroking their back to soothe them into sleep.

Bonding with your Newborn

Once you have brought the baby home, you will need to care for it over the next couple of months, until you return to work. These are crucial days; this is when the parents bond with the child the most. Obviously, this connection must be strengthened right away, or your baby's formative years will suffer.

It goes without saying that children thrive when the parents love them unconditionally – the best way to let your newborn know that is to cuddle with them. We have already discussed this previously, but I repeat it here to emphasize on its importance.

Cradle your newborn softly and gently stroke his/her back in repetitive, rhythmic patterns. This will not only allow for emotional bonding, it will also put them to sleep faster. Skin-to-skin contact with your baby, as in the Kangaroo Care, is a very effective method to show your child just how adored he/she is.

Babies love sounds; talk to your newborn and let them hear the sounds of your voice so that they slowly learn to recognize you, though open recognition will not happen for some time yet. Baby rattles and musical mobiles are also a good idea; they stimulate the baby's hearing. Sing your baby to sleep every night; you will be surprised at how much happier you and your baby will feel!

Some babies are extra sensitive to the light or noise; so if your child is, keep the lighting and noise levels dimmed so as to not startle them into crying.

Swaddling your Baby

This is a soothing technique that all new parents must learn. The baby's arms are close to the body while the legs are allowed to move; it keeps the child warm and gives them a sense of security and comfort. But swaddling can be tricky. Here is how you do it –

1. Spread a blanket out, with one corner folded over. Lay your baby face-up on it, head above the folded corner.

2. Wrap the left corner over your child; tuck it underneath the back of your newborn such that it goes under the arm

3. Pull the bottom corner over the feet and pull it up toward the head; fold it if it gets too close to the face. Don't make it too tight over the hips; leave it loose.

4. Wrap the right corner around the tiny form and then tuck it below his/her back on the left side. Only the neck and head should be left open. Slip a hand inside the blanket to make sure that it is not too tight or loose.

5. Remember, don't swaddle beyond 2 months. Infants start rolling around this time so stop swaddling.

Diapering

You should decide long before you give birth if you will use cloth or disposable diapers. Your baby will make you change its diapers at least 10 times a day, so be ready for that! Make sure that you have all your changing supplies before you start so that you don't leave your newborn unattended in the middle.

Lay the baby on their back and gently remove the wet diaper. With cotton balls, wash cloth and water, wipe the baby's genitals clean – wipe the bottom to avoid urinary tract infection. Apply ointment to heal a rash and always wash your hands before and after changing a diaper.

In case of rash, warm baths, diaper cream and some regular time away from diapers can help it heal better. If you use cloth diapers, then wash them in dye-free and fragrance-free detergents. If the rash persists for more than 3 days, then contact your doctor – he/she could be fighting an infection and may require medication.

Bathing

You should give your baby only a sponge bath until the umbilical cord falls off and the navel heals.

Initially, bathing your child 2-3 times a week is more than enough. Too many baths could hurt your baby's skin. Now, for a sponge bath, select a flat surface and fill a sink with lukewarm water.

Undress the baby and wrap him/her in a towel; wipe the baby's eyelids with a cotton ball or a soft wash cloth. Use another cotton ball for the other eye and then clean the nose and ears with a wash-cloth. The wet cloth and light baby soap to wash the rest of the baby carefully. Pat down gently to dry your baby with the towel and then dress him/her.

For tub baths, fill a small tub with lukewarm water and then place your baby inside; the water shouldn't more than 2-3 inches deep and don't let the tap run. Use one hand to support the head and the other to guide your baby in feet-first. Gently lower him/her into the tub up to the chest and wash the face/hair with a wash-cloth. Do the same with the rest of the body; remember to pour water regularly over them so that they don't get cold. Afterwards, wrap them in a towel instantly and cover the head.

Remember *never* leave the baby alone when bathing them. This is just asking for trouble.

Sleeping

Babies tend to sleep up to 16 hours in a day. Newborns sleep for 2-4 hours at a go, and then wake up, needing to be fed, changed or cuddled. Obviously, they won't let you sleep a full night; you'll have to wake up in the middle to feed or change them. Even if they don't wake up, you should wake them to feed them if they haven't eaten in more than 4 hours.

It's only when you hit the 3-month mark that your baby's sleep will begin to regularize. But again, there is no set pattern – like every pregnancy, every baby is different and each have their own sleep cycles and patterns. As long as they're healthy and gain the correct weight, don't worry too much about it; focus on working your sleeping patterns around your baby's to provide best care to both yourself and your child.

Remember to place your baby on its back to reduce risk of SIDS. Remove the fluffy quilts, bedding, toys and pillows and cushions from the crib so that he/she doesn't get tangled in them and then suffocate. Alternate the position of your newborns' head when you put him/her down each night, from left to right and then left again, so that they don't develop a flat spot on the head.

A good way to help your baby recognize that night-time is sleepy-time is to keep the stimulation at night at a minimum; use dim lighting and try to soothe him/her into sleep with lullabies and rocking motions. Reserve playing and fun for daytime so that they begin to understand that day is work and night is sleep.

As is obvious, there is a lot more to do when taking care of a newborn, but these are just the basics. Follow these guidelines to get started and do further research to make sure you know what you're doing! Always keep your doctor in the loop and don't be afraid to ask for advice! Talk to experts, talk to experienced friends and family so that you can give your baby the best possible care.

Conclusion

The information surrounding pregnancy and childcare given within this book is just the tip of the iceberg – it is only the barest minimum to get you started. Remember, there is no hard and fast rule that everything will happen as it's been described; every pregnancy is different and every child is unique. Even if you were to have ten children, there will be no two pregnancies alike and none of your children will be the same, even from birth!

Listen to your doctor's advice and keep in constant touch with those who have experienced these things previously. Physically and emotionally, pregnancy and childbirth are quite demanding of you as a woman, so don't be afraid to ask for help and take a break once in a while! Focus on keeping yourself healthy – you won't do your newborn much good if you run yourself ragged in the first week!

It's difficult, but it is also the most beautiful experience anyone can go through. Plan well, accept the challenges with a cheery attitude and take each day as it comes – enjoy your baby because it truly is a miracle!

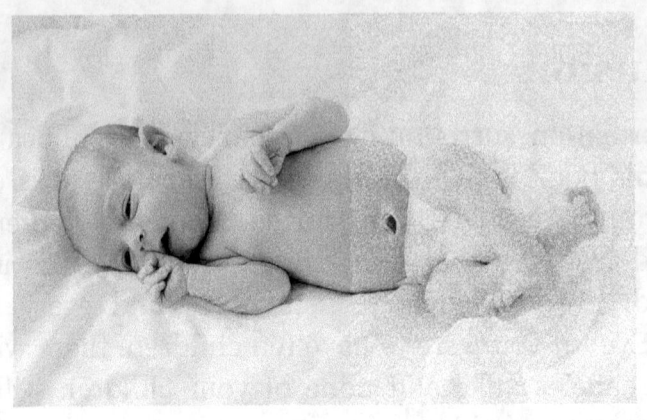

I hope you found this book informative and helpful! Thank you for choosing it!
Good luck with your bundle of joy!

Thank you for Reading! I Need Your Help...

Dear Reader,

I Hope you Enjoyed "**Pregnancy: Baby Smart, What You Need to Know to Start a Family - Motherhood, Childbirth & Nutrition**". I have to tell you, as an Author, I love feedback! I am always seeking ways to improve my current books and make the next ones better.

It's readers like you who have the biggest impact on a book's

success and development! So, tell me what you liked, what you

loved, and even what you hated. I would love to hear from you, and I

would like to ask you a favor, if you are so inclined, would you please

share a minute to review my book. Loved it, Hated it - I'd just enjoy

your feedback.

As you May have gleaned from my books, reviews can be tough to

come by these days and

You the reader have the power make or break the success of a book.

If you'd be so kind to

CLICK HERE to review the book, I would greatly appreciate it!

Thank you so much again for reading "**Pregnancy: Baby Smart,**

What You Need to Know to Start a Family - Motherhood,

Childbirth & Nutrition" and for spending time with me! I will see you

in the next one!

Check Out More From The Publisher...

Psychology: Hypnosis & Mind Control – To Overcome Stress, Anxiety,
Depression & Finally Recover Your Happiness
by Fred McGaughy
http://www.amazon.com/Psychology-Hypnosis-Depression-Happiness-
Brainwashing-ebook/dp/B014AMVA3E

Paleo: The Ultimate Paleo Mass Gain Plan: How to Add Muscle and Gain

Weight on the Paleo Diet
by John Grokowski
http://www.amazon.com/Paleo-Workout-Supplement-Building-Crossfit-ebook/dp/B01573FAIG

Marriage: Romance Your Mate Again, With Spicy Sex Secrets, Pleasure, Taboo And Sex Positions that will Blow Their Mind
by Veronica Counsel
http://www.amazon.com/Marriage-Pleasure-Positions-Intimacy-Counseling-ebook/dp/B016SGTEY2

Gut: The Key to Ultimate Health - SIBO, IBS & Fatigue
by Maria Lexington
http://www.amazon.com/Healthy-Living-Happiness-Schizophrenia-Fibromyalgia-ebook/dp/B010KM9CLA

Krav Maga: Dominating Solutions to Real World Violence
by George Silva
http://www.amazon.com/Krav-Maga-Dominating-Solutions-Violence-ebook/dp/B01A2BL6CW